The Super Tasty Ketogenic Recipe Guide

*Healthy and Tasty Ketogenic Recipes to Enjoy
Your Diet and Boost Your Taste*

Lauren Loose

Contents

Egg-Crust Pizza

Preparation Time: 5 minutes

Cooking Time: 15 minutes

Servings: 2

Ingredients

- ¼ teaspoon of dried oregano to taste
- ½ teaspoon of spike seasoning to taste
- 1 ounce of mozzarella, chopped into small cubes
- 6 – 8 sliced thinly black olives
- 6 slices of turkey pepperoni, sliced into half
- 4-5 thinly sliced small grape tomatoes
- 2 eggs, beaten well
- 1-2 teaspoons of olive oil

Directions

1. Preheat the broiler in an oven than in a small bowl, beat well the eggs. Cut the pepperoni and tomatoes in slices then cut the mozzarella cheese into cubes.

2. Drizzle oil in a skillet at medium heat, then heat the pan for around one minute until it begins to get hot. Add in eggs and season with oregano and spike seasoning, then cook for around 2 minutes.

3. Drizzle half of the mozzarella, olives, pepperoni, and tomatoes on the eggs followed by another layer of the remaining half of the above ingredients. Ensure that there is a lot of cheese on the topmost layers. Cover and cook for 4 minutes.

4. Position the pan under the preheated broiler and cook until the top has browned and the cheese has melted nicely for around 2-3 minutes. Serve immediately.

Nutrition

363 Calories

24.1g Fats

20.8g Carbohydrates

Breakfast Roll-Ups

Preparation Time: 5 minutes

Cooking Time: 15 minutes

Servings: 5

Ingredients

- Non-stick cooking spray
- 5 patties of cooked breakfast sausage
- 5 slices of cooked bacon
- cups of cheddar cheese, shredded
- Pepper and salt
- 10 large eggs

Directions

1. Prep a skillet on medium to high heat, then using a whisk, combine two of the eggs in a mixing bowl.
2. After the pan has become hot, lower the heat to medium-low heat then put in the eggs. If you want to, you can utilize some cooking spray.
3. Season eggs with some pepper and salt.
4. Seal the eggs and leave them to cook for a couple of minutes or until the eggs are almost cooked.

5. Drizzle around 1/3 cup of cheese on top of the eggs, then place a strip of bacon and divide the sausage into two and place on top.

6. Roll the egg carefully on top of the fillings. The roll-up will almost look like a taquitos. If you have a hard time folding over the egg, use a spatula to keep the egg intact until the egg has molded into a roll-up.

7. Put aside the roll-up then repeat the above steps until you have four more roll-ups; you should have 5 roll-ups in total.

Nutrition:

412.2g Calories

31.6g Fats

2.26g Carbohydrates

Basic Opie Rolls

Preparation Time: 20 minutes

Cooking Time: 35 minutes

Servings: 12

Ingredients

- 1/8 teaspoon of salt
- 1/8 teaspoon of cream of tartar
- 3 ounces of cream cheese
- 3 large eggs

Direction

1. Prepare oven to about 300 degrees, then separate the egg whites from egg yolks and place both eggs in different bowls. Using an electric mixer, beat well the egg whites until the mixture is very bubbly, then stir in the cream of tartar and mix.

2. In the bowl with the egg yolks, put in 3 ounces of cubed cheese and salt. Mix well until the mixture has doubled in size and is pale yellow. Put in the egg white mixture into the egg yolk mixture then fold the mixture gently together.

3. Spray some oil on the cookie sheet coated with some parchment paper, then add dollops of the batter and bake for around 30 minutes.

4. You will know they are ready when the upper part of the rolls is firm and golden. Put aside on a wire rack. Enjoy with some coffee.

Nutrition:

45 Calories

4g Fats

2g Proteins

Almond Coconut Egg Wraps

Preparation time: 5 minutes

Cooking time: 5 minutes

Servings: 4

Ingredients:

- 5 Organic eggs
- 1 tbsp. Coconut flour
- 25 tsp. Sea salt
- 2 tbsp. almond meal

Directions:

1. Combine the fixings in a blender and work them until creamy. Heat a skillet using the med-high temperature setting.
2. Fill two tablespoons of batter into the skillet and cook - covered about three minutes. Turn it over to cook for another 3 minutes. Serve the wraps piping hot.

Nutrition:

3g Carbohydrates

8g Protein

111 Calories

Bacon & Avocado Omelet

Preparation Time: 5 minutes

Cooking Time: 5 minutes

Servings: 1

Ingredients:

- 1 slice Crispy bacon
- 2 Large organic eggs
- 5 cup freshly grated parmesan cheese
- 2 tbsp. Ghee or coconut oil or butter
- half of 1 small Avocado

Directions:

1. Prepare the bacon to your liking and set aside. Combine the eggs, parmesan cheese, and your choice of finely chopped herbs. Warm a skillet and add the butter/ghee to melt using the medium-high heat setting. When the pan is hot, whisk and add the eggs.

2. Prepare the omelet working it towards the middle of the pan for about 30 seconds. When firm, flip, and cook it for another 30 seconds. Arrange the omelet on a plate and garnish with the crunched bacon bits. Serve with sliced avocado.

Nutrition:

3.3g Carbohydrates

30g Protein

719 Calories

Bacon & Cheese Frittata

Preparation Time: 5 minutes

Cooking Time: 5 minutes

Servings: 6

Ingredients:

- 1 cup Heavy cream
- 6 Eggs
- 5 Crispy slices of bacon
- 2 Chopped green onions
- 4 oz. Cheddar cheese

Directions:

1. Warm the oven temperature to reach 350º Fahrenheit.
2. Scourge eggs and seasonings. Fill into the pie pan and top off with the remainder of the fixings. Bake 30-35 minutes. Wait for a few minutes before serving for best results.

Nutrition:

2g Carbohydrates

13g Protein

320 Calories

Bacon & Egg Breakfast Muffins

Preparation Time: 15 minutes

Cooking Time: 30 minutes

Servings: 12

Ingredients:

- 8 large Eggs
- 8 slices Bacon
- .66 cup Green onion

Directions:

1. Warm the oven at 350° Fahrenheit. Spritz the muffin tin wells using a cooking oil spray. Chop the onions and set aside.

2. Prepare a large skillet using the medium temperature setting. Fry the bacon until it's crispy and place on a layer of paper towels to drain the grease. Chop it into small pieces after it has cooled.

3. Whisk the eggs, bacon, and green onions, mixing well until all of the fixings are incorporated. Dump the egg mixture into the muffin tin (halfway full). Bake it for about 20 to 25 minutes. Cool slightly and serve.

Nutrition:

0.4g Carbohydrates

5.6g Protein

69 Calories

Bacon Hash

Preparation Time: 5 minutes

Cooking Time: 10 minutes

Servings: 2

Ingredients:

- 1 Small green pepper
- 2 Jalapenos
- 1 Small onion
- 4 Eggs
- 6 Bacon slices

Directions:

1. Chop the bacon into chunks using a food processor. Set aside for now. Cut onions and peppers into thin strips. Dice the jalapenos as small as possible.
2. Heat a skillet and fry the veggies. Once browned, combine the fixings and cook until crispy. Place on a serving dish with the eggs.

Nutrition:

9g Carbohydrates

23g Protein

366 Calories

Grilled Peppered Steaks

Preparation Time: 5 minutes

Cooking Time: 15 minutes

Serving: 4

Ingredients

- 2 teaspoons coarsely ground pepper
- 1 teaspoon onion salt
- 1 teaspoon garlic salt
- 1/4 teaspoon paprika
- 4 boneless beef top loin steaks

Direction:

1. Mix the pepper, onion salt, garlic salt, and, if desired, paprika. Rub onto both steaks.
2. Grill, sealed, over moderate heat until meat reaches ideal doneness (for medium-rare, a thermometer should read One35°; medium, 140°; medium-well, 145°) 10 minutes on each side.

Nutrition

10g fat

301 calories

1g carbohydrate

Buffalo Pulled Chicken

Preparation Time: 10 minutes

Cooking Time: 4 hours

Serving: 4

Ingredients

- 2 cup Buffalo wing sauce
- 2tablespoons ranch salad dressing mix
- 4 chicken breast halves (6 ounces each)

Direction:

1. Using 3-qt. slow cooker, mix wing sauce, and dressing mix. Cook chicken on low for 4 hours.
2. Shred chicken with two forks. Serve with celery, top with additional wing sauce and cheese, and serve with ranch dressing.

Nutrition

147 calories

3g fat

6g carbohydrate

Italian Smothered Pork Chops

Preparation Time: 10 minutes

Cooking Time: 30 minutes

Serving: 4

Ingredients

- 2-pound broccoli rabe
- 4boneless pork loin chops
- 1 teaspoon salt
- 1 teaspoon garlic powder
- 2 teaspoon pepper
- 1tablespoon canola oil
- 2 cup sliced roasted sweet red pepper
- 4 ounces fresh mozzarella cheese

Direction:

1. Preheat broiler. Trim 2 broccoli rabe; discard any coarse leaves.
2. Bring 4 cups of water to a large saucepan. Boil broccoli rabe uncovered, 5 minutes. Remove and immediately drop into ice water. Pat dry.
3. Sprinkle pork chops with seasonings, in a broiler-safe skillet, heat oil at medium-high heat. Cook pork chops for 8 minutes on both sides. Remove from heat.

4. Layer chops with red pepper, broccoli rabe, and cheese. Broil 4 from heat for 2 minutes.

Nutrition

365 calories

20g fat

4g carbohydrate

Pistachio Salmon

Preparation Time: 10 minutes

Cooking Time: 20 minutes

Serving: 1

Ingredients

- 1/3 cup pistachios, finely chopped
- 1/4 cup panko bread crumbs
- 1/4 cup grated Parmesan cheese
- 1 salmon fillet (One pound)
- 1/2 teaspoon salt
- 1/4 teaspoon pepper

Direction:

1. Preheat oven to 400°F. Toss pistachios with bread crumbs and cheese.
2. Place salmon on a greased foil-lined in. Pan, skin side down; season. Top with pistachio mixture, pressing to adhere. Bake, uncovered, for 20 minutes.

Nutrition

458 calories

6.8 g carbohydrates

36.2g protein

Pan-Roast Chicken

Preparation Time: 10 minutes

Cooking Time: 1 hour

Serving: 4

Ingredient

- 1 fryer chicken (5 pounds)
- 2 teaspoons kosher salt
- 1teaspoon coarsely ground pepper
- 2 teaspoons olive oil
- Minced fresh thyme or rosemary, optional

Direction:

1. Rub outside of the chicken with salt and pepper. Transfer chicken to a rack on a rimmed baking sheet. Refrigerate, uncovered, overnight.
2. Preheat oven to 450°. Remove chicken from refrigerator while oven heats. Preheat 12-inch cast-iron skillet in the oven for 15 minutes.
3. Place chicken on a work surface, neck side down. Cut through the skin where legs connect to the body. Press thighs down so joints pop and legs lie flat.
4. Carefully place chicken into hot skillet; breast side up and press legs down. Brush with oil. Roast for 40 minutes. Remove chicken from

oven; let stand 10 minutes. Top with herbs before serving.

Nutrition

24g fat

405 calories

44g protein.

Bacon-Wrapped Spam Bites

Preparation Time: 5 minutes

Cooking Time: 15 minutes

Serving: 6

Ingredients

- 16 bacon strips
- 1 can (12 ounces) reduced-sodium SPAM, cut into 12 cubes
- 1/3 cup yellow mustard
- 1/4 cup maple syrup
- 1 garlic clove

Direction:

1. Preheat oven to 400°. Cut bacon strips crosswise in half. Fry bacon over moderate heat in a large skillet. Remove to drain to paper towels.

2. Wrap a piece of bacon around every cube of Spam; secure it with a toothpick. Place in a 15x10x1-in. ungreased baking pan. Bake for 10 minutes. Mix mustard, syrup, and garlic; drizzle over bacon-wrapped Spam. Bake for 10 minutes.

Nutrition

60 calories

4g fat

2g carbohydrate

Southern Pimiento Cheese Spread

Preparation Time: 10 minutes

Cooking Time: 0 minute

Serving: 4

Ingredients

- 1 ½ cups shredded cheddar cheese
- 1 jar (4 ounces) diced pimientos
- 1/3 cup mayonnaise
- Assorted crackers

Directions

1. Combine cheese, pimientos, and mayonnaise. Refrigerate for at least 1 hour. Serve with crackers.

Nutrition

11g fat

116 calories

1g carbohydrate

Cod and Asparagus Bake

Preparation Time: 5 minutes

Cooking Time: 15 minutes

Serving: 4

Ingredients

- 4 cod fillets (4 ounces each)
- 1-pound fresh thin asparagus
- 1-pint cherry tomatoes halved
- 2 tablespoons lemon juice
- 1 ½ teaspoons grated lemon zest
- 1/4 cup grated Romano cheese

Direction:

1. Preheat oven to 375 degrees. Place asparagus and cod in a 15x10x1-in. Baking pan brushed with oil. Add tomatoes, cut sides down. Brush fish with lemon juice; sprinkle with lemon zest.
2. Sprinkle fish and vegetables with Romano cheese. Bake for 12minutes.
3. Remove from oven; preheat broiler—broil cod mixture 4 inch from heat for 3 minutes.

Nutrition

141 calories

3g fat

6g carbohydrates

Sautéed Garlic Mushrooms

Preparation Time: 10 minutes

Cooking Time: 5 minutes

Serving: 5

Ingredients

- 3/4 pound sliced fresh mushrooms
- 3 teaspoons minced garlic
- 1 tablespoon seasoned bread crumb
- 1/3 cup butter, cubed

Direction:

1. Sauté the mushrooms, garlic, and bread crumbs in butter in a large skillet until the mushrooms get tender.

Nutrition

177 Calories

5g Carbohydrates

2g Protein

Sautéed Radishes with Green Beans

Preparation Time: 5 minutes

Cooking Time: 5 minutes

Serving: 3

Ingredients

- 1 tablespoon butter
- ½ pound fresh green or wax beans, trimmed
- 1 cup thinly sliced radishes
- ½ teaspoon sugar
- 1/4 teaspoon salt
- 2 tablespoons pine nuts, toasted

Direction:

1. In a huge skillet, melt butter over medium-high heat. Cook beans for 4 minutes.
2. Cook radishes for 3 minutes longer stirring rarely. Mix in sugar and salt; sprinkle with nuts.

Nutrition

75 calories

6g fat

5g carbohydrate

Easy Ketogenic Smoked Salmon Lunch Bowl

Preparation Time: 10 minutes

Cooking Time: 5 minutes

Serving: 2

Ingredients

- 12-ounce smoked salmon
- 4 tablespoon mayonnaise
- 2-ounce spinach
- 1 tablespoon olive oil
- ½ medium lime

Direction:

1. Arrange the mayonnaise, salmon, spinach on a plate.
2. Sprinkle olive oil over the spinach.
3. Serve with lime wedges and Season with salt and pepper.

Nutrition

457 calories

1.9g carbohydrates

34.8g fats

Easy One-Pan Ground Beef and Green Beans

Preparation Time: 10 minutes

Cooking Time: 15 minutes

Serving: 2

Ingredients

- 10 ounces (80/20) ground beef
- 9 ounces green beans
- 2 tablespoons sour cream
- 3½ ounces butter

Direction

1. Wash the green beans, then trim the ends off each side.
2. Put half of the butter to a pan over high heat.
3. Once hot, put the ground beef and season. Cook the beef until it's almost done.
4. Decrease heat on the pan to medium. Add the remaining butter and the green beans to the pan and cook for 5 minutes. Stir the ground beef and green beans occasionally.
5. Season the green beans. Serve with a dollop of sour cream.

Nutrition

787.5 Calories

71.75g Fats

27.5g Protein.

Easy Spinach and Bacon Salad

Preparation Time: 5 minutes

Cooking Time: 5 minutes

Serving: 4

Ingredients

- 8 ounces spinach
- 4 large hard-boiled eggs
- 6 ounces bacon
- 1/2 medium red onion
- 1/2 cup mayonnaise

Direction:

1. Pan-fry bacon until it is done and crispy. Chop into pieces once cooked and set aside.
2. Slice the hard-boiled eggs and, rinse the spinach.
3. Combine the lettuce, mayonnaise, and remaining bacon fat into a large cup season.
4. Toss red onion, sliced eggs, and bacon into the salad. Serve immediately.

Nutrition

45.9g Fats

509.15 Calories

19.75g Protein

Easy Ketogenic Italian Plate

Preparation Time: 5 minutes

Cooking Time: 0 minute

Serving: 4

Ingredients

- 7 ounces fresh mozzarella cheese
- 7 ounces prosciutto
- 2 medium tomatoes
- 4 tablespoons olive oil
- 10 whole green olives

Direction:

1. Arrange the tomato, olives, mozzarella, and prosciutto on a plate.
2. Season the tomato and cheese. Serve with olive oil.

Nutrition

780.9 Calories

5.9g Carbohydrates

60.74g Fats

Fresh Broccoli and Dill
Ketogenic Salad

Preparation Time: 10 minutes

Cooking Time: 5 minutes

Serving: 3

Ingredients

- 16 ounces broccoli
- 1/2 cup mayonnaise
- 3/4 cup chopped fresh dill

Direction:

1. Chop the broccoli into small pieces. Cut the stems into even smaller pieces.
2. Boil salted water. Boil broccoli to the pot for 5 minutes. Drain the broccoli and set aside.
3. Once cooled, add the remaining ingredients and stir together. Season, serve afterward.

Nutrition

303.3 Calories

28.1g Fats

4.03g Protein

Bulletproof Chocolate Smoothie

Preparation Time: 3 minutes

Cooking Time: 2 minutes

Servings 2

Ingredients:

- 1 ¼ cup fresh brewed coffee, cooled for at least 15 minutes
- ¼ cup filtered water
- 2 scoops Chocolate Collagen Protein Powder
- 6-8 Ice cubes

Directions:

1. Blend coffee, water and chocolate protein powder until smooth, adding ice cubes until you reach desired consistency.
2. Serve right away.

Nutrition:

30 Calories

1g Fat

Basic Bulletproof Coffee Drink

Preparation Time: 2 minutes

Cooking Time: 1 minute

Servings 1

Ingredients:

- 1 cup brewed coffee
- 1 tsp. coconut oil
- 1 tbsp. butter, unsalted
- ¼ tsp. vanilla extract
- A few drops of stevia

Directions:

1. Put all ingredients into blender. Pulse on high for 20 seconds until frothy. Drink immediately.

Nutrition:

148 Calories

14g Fat

Strawberry Avocado Green Smoothie

Preparation Time: 5 minutes

Cooking Time: 5 minutes

Servings: 2

Ingredients:

- 1 cup fresh strawberries, hulled
- ½ medium, ripe avocado, peeled
- 1 cup (packed) baby spinach
- 1 cup unsweetened almond milk
- 2 teaspoons sweetener
- 6-8 ice cubes

Direction:

1. Position all ingredients into blender and blend until smooth. Once blended, taste for sweetness and adjust accordingly by adding more strawberries or sweetener as needed. Serve immediately.

Nutrition:

156 Calories

6.9g Fat

2.7g Protein

Peanut Butter Cup Smoothie

Preparation Time 5 minutes

Cooking Time: 0 minute

Servings 2

Ingredients:

- 1 cup water
- ¾ cup coconut cream
- 1 scoop chocolate protein powder
- 2 tablespoons natural peanut butter
- 3 ice cubes

Directions:

1. Put the water, coconut cream, protein powder, peanut butter and ice in a blender and blend until smooth. Pour into 2 glasses and serve immediately.

Nutrition:

486 Calories

40g Fat

30g Protein

Berry Green Smoothie

Preparation Time 10 minutes

Cooking Time: 0 minute

Servings: 2

Ingredients:

- 1 cup water
- ½ cup raspberries
- ½ cup shredded kale
- ¾ cup cream cheese
- 1 tablespoon coconut oil
- 1 scoop vanilla protein powder

Directions:

1. Put the water, raspberries, kale, cream cheese, coconut oil and protein powder in a blender and blend until smooth. Pour into 2 glasses and serve immediately.

Nutrition:

436 Calories

36g Fat

28g Protein

Green banana pancakes

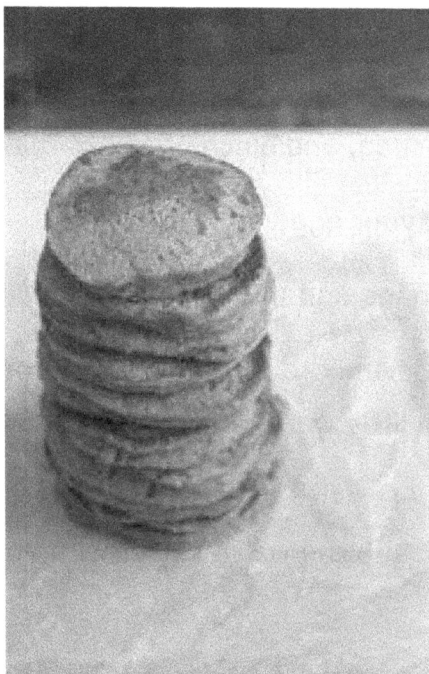

Total time: 20 minutes

Ingredients:

2 large peeled bananas

2 eggs

6 tablespoons of coconut flour

2 teaspoons cassava flour or arrowroot starch

Pinch of salt

¼ teaspoon stevia powder

1 tablespoon of baking powder

Coconut oil or grass-fed butter

Directions

Mash the banana till its smooth

In another bowl, mix the coconut flour, stevia, arrowroot, or cassava, baking soda, and pinch of salt to make a powder mix

Crack and whisk your egg very lightly.

Pour into the banana and mix up

Pour in the powder mix to the banana and egg [If the mix is too thick, pour in little water at a time. Use a spoon to pour in water.]

Preheat a skillet. Rub the warm skillet with your butter, ghee, or oil.

Pour in your batter to the skillet with a spoon

When it is golden brown on the outside, flip it and let it cool

Serve warm

Berry bread spread

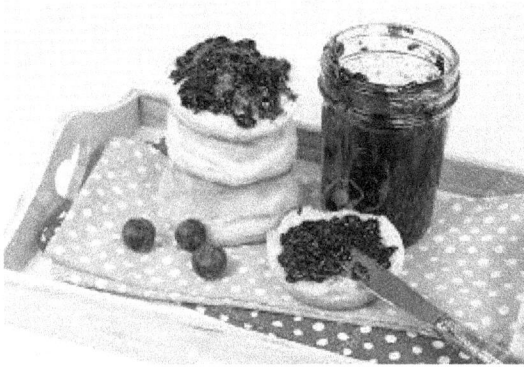

Total time : 15 minutes

Ingredients :

2 cups of coconut cream

2 ounces of strawberries

1 ½ ounces of blueberries

1 ½ ounces of raspberries

½ teaspoon coconut extract

Directions

Separate 3 of each berry type and dice in small pieces

Put in the strawberries, blueberries, and raspberries in a blender till its smooth

Pour out and mix with coconut extract and coconut cream

Mix till smooth and blend again

Pour in diced berries

Serve

48

Chocolate bread spread

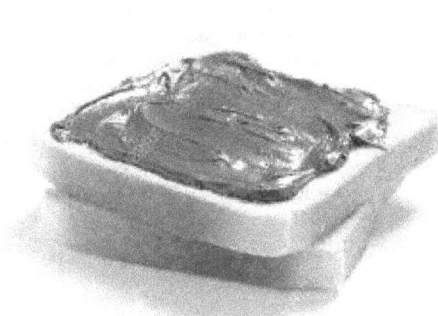

Total time: 20 minutes

Ingredients :

4 cups of sweet cream

2 ounces of coconut oil

3 ounces of chocolate

1 teaspoon of coconut extract

1 tablespoon of powdered cacao

Groundnuts [optional]

Directions

Place sweet cream in a microwavable bowl and heat for 10-15 seconds

Pour in coconut oil and stir

Put in chocolate and cacao

Put in microwave for a little under a minute

When it is warm, you can put in your groundnuts if you want them in

Place in bowls and refrigerate

Ketogenic almond cereal

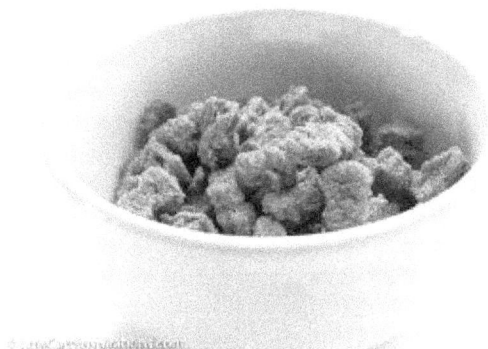

Total time: 25 minutes

Ingredients :

3 cups of unsweetened coconut flakes

1 cup of sliced almonds

¾ tablespoon of cinnamon

¾ tablespoon of nutmeg

Directions

Preheat oven to 250 degrees F

The almonds and coconut flakes together

Pour in the nutmeg and cinnamon

Put on a baking tray at bake for 3-5 minutes

Depending on the thickness of your coconut, it can be ready sooner. Take off when slightly brown

Enjoy with milk

Ketogenic granola cereal

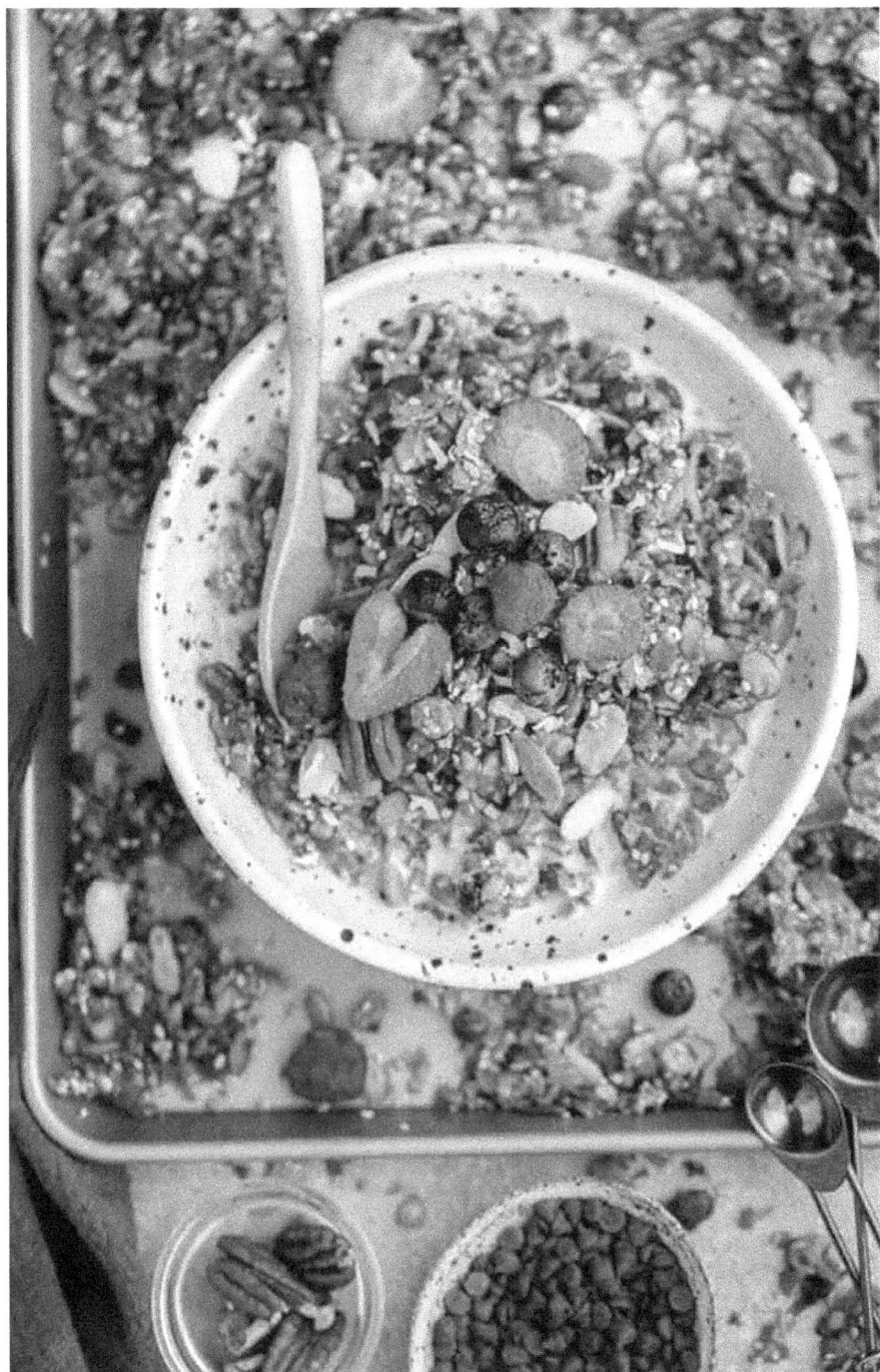

Total time: 35 minutes

Ingredients :

1 cup of flaxseeds

Directions

Beat the egg

Preheat oven to 300 degrees F

Set out a bowl and put in all ingredients

Set out a baking pan with parchment paper

Pour ingredients in

Bake for 30 minutes

Ketogenic fruit cereal

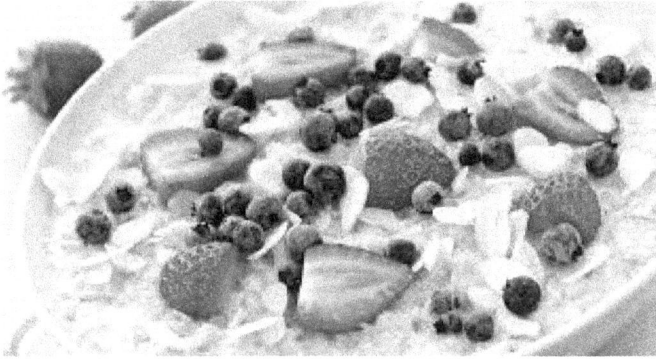

Total time: 25 minutes

Ingredients :

1 cup of coconut flakes

½ cup of sliced strawberries

¼ cup of sliced raspberries

Directions

Preheat oven to 300 degrees F

Set out a baking pan with parchment paper

Pour the flakes in

Bake for 5 minutes

Pour in sliced raspberries and strawberries.

Enjoy with almond milk

Ketogenic chicken and avocado

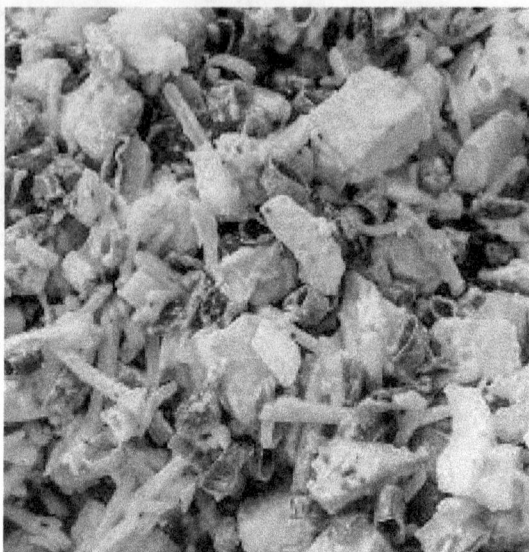

Total time: 25 minutes

Ingredients :

6 medium-sized pieces of chicken. Boneless.

1 avocado

2 eggs

Ketogenic Mayo

Salt

 Pepper

Ground Garlic

1/8 cup of olive oil

Directions

Soft boil 2 eggs

Put the seasonings together in a bowl

Sprinkle them generously on the chicken.

Cover for 5 minutes

Heat up the olive oil and fry the chicken

Take out the chicken and set aside

Cut avocado in two and remove the pit

Dice on half and set aside

Slice the eggs in half so you have four pieces

Sprinkle a little salt on the avocados [optional]

Spread mayo on the chicken [optional]

On a place, set your eggs, meat, and avocados. Enjoy warm

Ketogenic almond pancake

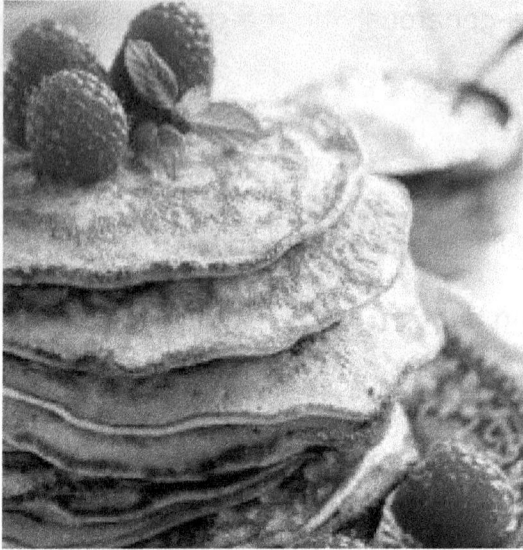

Total time: 30 minutes

Ingredients :

1 ½ cups of almond flour

3 teaspoons of baking powder

1 teaspoon of salt

1 tablespoon of stevia

1 ¼ cup of almond milk

1 egg

3 tablespoons of melted ghee

2 teaspoons of olive oil

Directions

Put in dry ingredients and stir.

In another bowl, mix egg and mix

Pour the wet inside the dry and add the butter.

Mix well

Heat a frying pan and

Pour in olive oil to the pot at teaspoon at a time

Pour in the batter and brown each side equally

Serve warm

Ketogenic meat balls

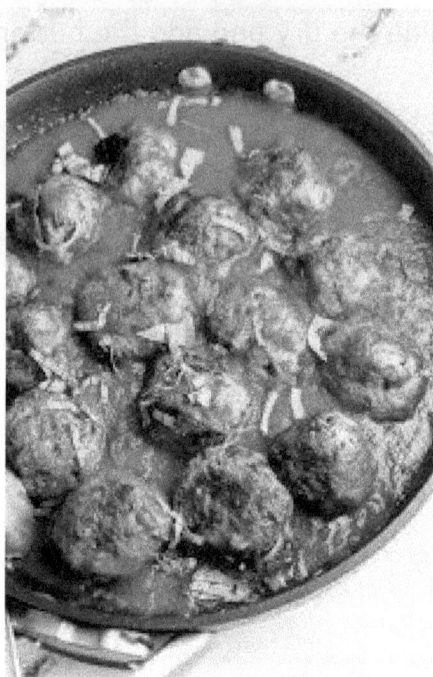

Total time: 35 minutes

Ingredients :

11 eggs

7 ounces of mozzarella cheese

4 ounces of chopped and cooked bacon

3 chopped scallions

1 ounce of ground beef

Salt

Pepper

Teaspoon of olive oil

Directions

Preheat oven to 350 degrees F

Spray baking spray on your muffin tin

Put the scallions evenly in the tin. Let them be at the bottom

In a bowl, mix eggs and add a teaspoon of oil

Pour in cheese and add salt and pepper to taste.

In another bowl, mix bacon and chicken

Pour it into cheese and stir

Pour the mix into the tray and bake for 17-20 minutes

Ketogenic scrambled eggs

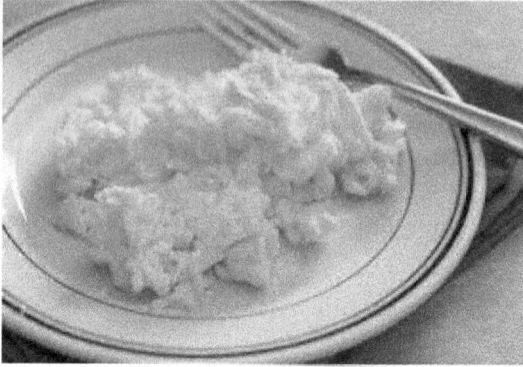

Total time: 15 minutes

Ingredients :

3 eggs

1 ounce of ghee

Salt and pepper

Directions

Crack eggs and mix with salt and pepper

Heat skillet and pour in butter'

When slightly melted, pour in eggs and scramble

Banana Waffles

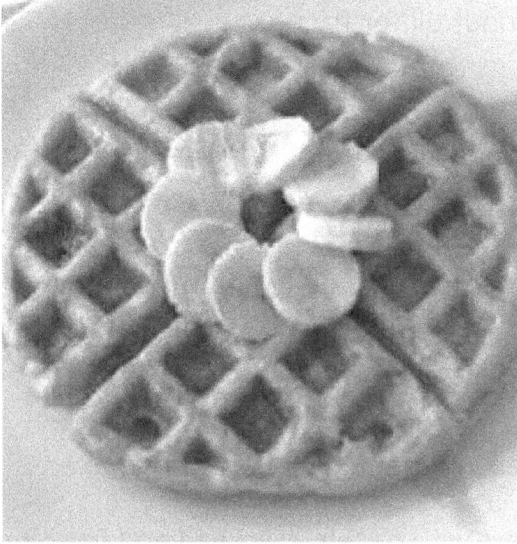

Total time: 35 minutes

Ingredients :

4 eggs

1 ripe banana

¾ cup coconut milk

¾ cup almond flour

1 pinch of salt

1 tbsp. of ground psyllium husk powder

½ tsp. vanilla extract

1 tsp. baking powder

1 tsp. of ground cinnamon

Butter or coconut oil for frying

Directions:

Mash the banana thoroughly until you get a mashed potato consistency.

Add all the other ingredients in and whisk thoroughly to evenly distribute the dry and wet ingredients. You should be able to get a pancake-like consistency

Fry the waffles in a pan or use a waffle maker.

You can serve it with hazelnut spread and fresh berries. Enjoy!

Ketogenic Cinnamon Coffee

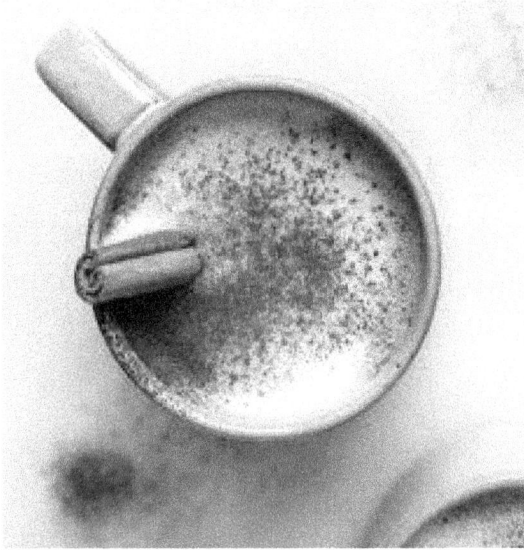

Total time: 10 minutes

Ingredients :

2 tbsp. ground coffee

1/3 cup heavy whipping cream

1 tsp. ground cinnamon

2 cups water

Directions:

Start by mixing the cinnamon with the ground coffee.

Pour in hot water and do what you usually do when brewing.

Use a mixer or whisk to whip the cream 'til you get stiff peaks

Serve in a tall mug and put the whipped cream on the surface. Sprinkle with some cinnamon and enjoy.

Ketogenic Waffles and Blueberries

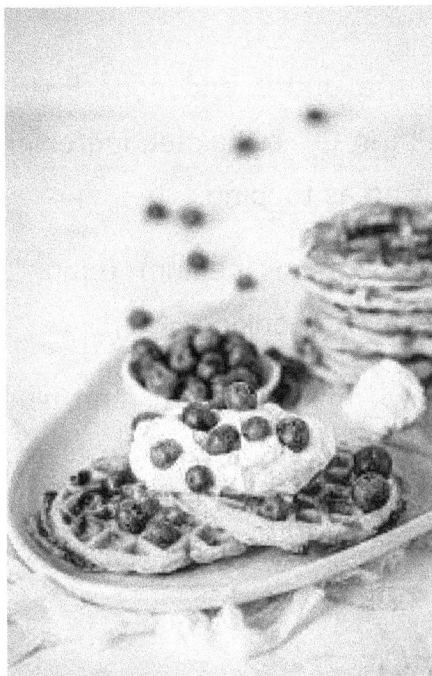

Total time: 20 minutes

Ingredients :

8 eggs

5 oz. melted butter

1 tsp. vanilla extract

2 tsp. baking powder

1/3 cup coconut flour

3 oz. butter (topping)

1 oz. fresh blueberries (topping)

Directions:

Start by mixing the butter and eggs first until you get a smooth batter. Put in the remaining ingredients except those that we will be using as topping.

Heat your waffle iron to medium temperature and start pouring in the batter for cooking

In a separate bowl, mix the butter and blueberries using a hand mixer. Use this to top off your freshly cooked waffles

Baked Avocado Eggs

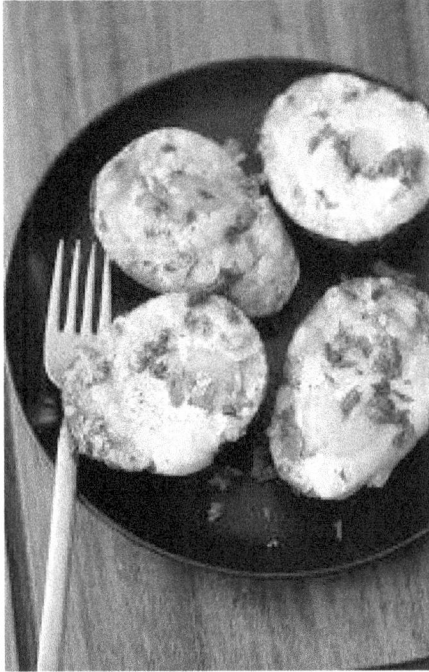

Total time: 35 minutes

Ingredients :

2 avocados

4 eggs

½ cup bacon bits, around 55 grams

2 tbsp. fresh chives, chopped

1 sprig of chopped fresh basil, chopped

1 cherry tomato, quartered

Salt and pepper to taste

Shredded cheddar cheese

Directions:

Start by preheating the oven to 400 degrees Fahrenheit

Slice the avocado and remove the pits. Put them on a baking sheet and crack some eggs onto the center hole of the avocado. If it is too small, just scoop out more of the flesh to make room. Salt and pepper to taste.

Top with bacon bits and bake for 15 minutes.

Remove and sprinkle with herbs. Enjoy!

Mushroom Omelet

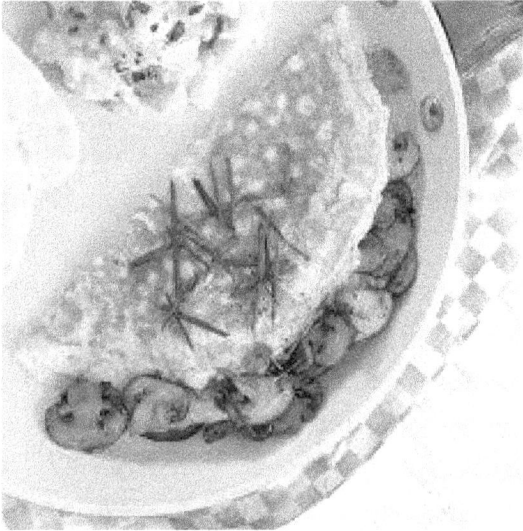

Total time: 10 minutes

Ingredients :

3 eggs, medium

1 oz. shredded cheese

1 oz. butter used for frying

¼ yellow onion, chopped

4 large sliced mushrooms

Your favorite vegetables, optional

Salt and pepper to taste

Directions:

Crack and whisk the eggs in a bowl. Add some salt and pepper to taste.

Melt the butter in a pan using low heat. Put in the mushroom and onion, cooking the two until you get that amazing smell.

Pour the egg mix into the pan and allow it to cook on medium heat.

Allow the bottom part to cook before sprinkling the cheese on top of the still-raw portion of the egg.

Carefully pry the edges of the omelet and fold it in half. Allow it to cook for a few more seconds before removing the pan from the heat and sliding it directly onto your plate.

Soft Boiled Ketogenic Eggs

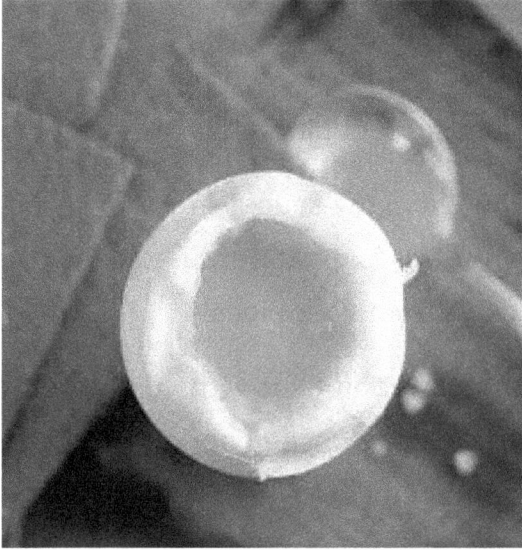

Total time: 20 minutes

Ingredients :

3 large eggs

1 tbsp. of unsalted butter

¼ tsp. thyme leaves

Freshly ground black pepper

Salt to taste

Directions:

Grab a saucepan and fill it halfway with water, apply high heat until the water boils.

When boiling, gently place the eggs in the water. Set a timer for 6 minutes.

Take on tablespoon of butter and put it in the microwave for around 20 seconds or until it melts.

Remove the eggs from the saucepan, carefully pouring the hot water in the sink. This is great because the hot water can also help remove clogs from your pipes!

Carefully take a bowl and fill it with cold water. Put the eggs inside so it can cool off. Once done, peel the egg and place it in your bowl of melted butter.

Add salt and pepper to taste and thyme for garnishing. Make sure to eat it while fresh!

French Omelet

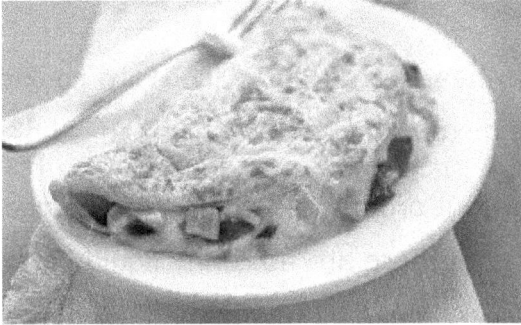

Total time: 30 minutes

Ingredients :

2 large eggs

4 large egg whites

¼ cup fat-free milk

¼ cup cubed ham, cooked

¼ cup cheddar cheese, shredded

1/8 tsp. salt

1/8 tsp. pepper

1 tbsp. onion, chopped

1 tbsp. green pepper, chopped

Directions:

Whisk together the eggs and egg whites until blended.

Add the salt, pepper, and milk, mixing them together until fully blended.

Using medium heat, coat your skillet with cooking spray and pour the egg mixture in when the surface is hot and ready.

As it cooks, push it around the edges so the uncooked portion flows around until there are no runny liquid on top.

When it is already around ¾ cooked, put all the remaining ingredients on top and continue cooking until done.

Apple Chicken Sausage

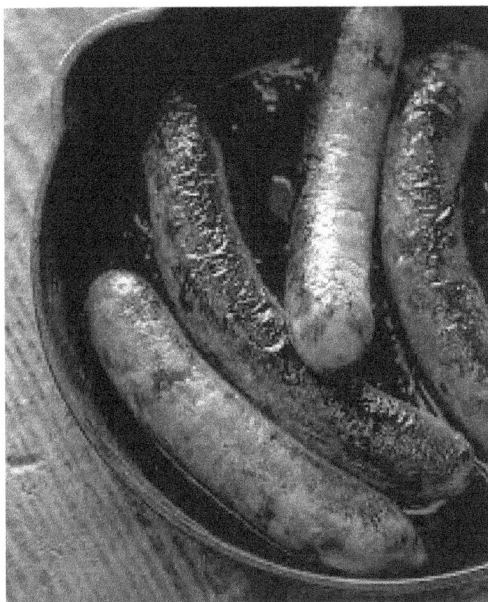

Total time: 35 minutes

Ingredients :

1 large tart apple, diced

1-pound ground chicken

¼ tsp. pepper

1 tsp. salt

2 tsp. poultry seasoning

Directions:

Grab a large bowl and combine all the ingredients except the ground chicken

Combine the chicken in the mix and blend well. Create a total of 8 patties of similar sizes which should be around 3 inches in diameter each.

Cook them up using medium heat. Make sure each side gets around 5 to 6 minutes of cooking time.

Ketogenic Cereal

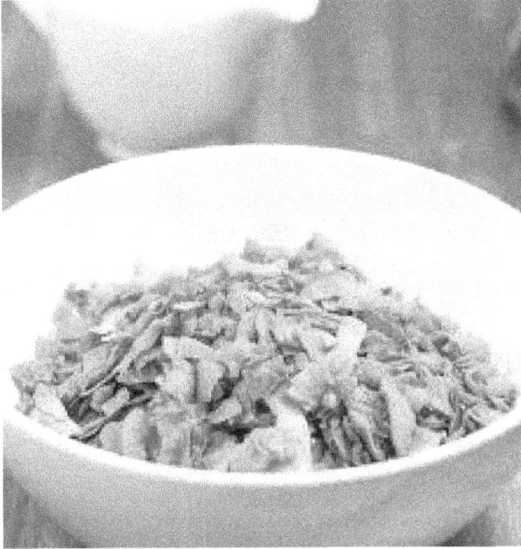

Total time: 1 hours 20 minutes

Ingredients :

1 cup shredded coconut, unsweetened

1 cup flaked coconut, unsweetened

½ cup flaxseeds

½ cup flaked almonds

1/3 cup Pepitas

1/3 cup sunflower seeds

1/3 cup chia seeds

1/3 cup erythritol

1/3 cup melted coconut oil

1 tbsp. ground cinnamon

1 tsp. vanilla extract

Directions:

Preheat your over to 150 degrees Celsius or 300 degrees Fahrenheit

Mix all the ingredients together in one convenient bowl.

Once they are combined, spread them over a pan on top of a lined cookie sheet

Bake them for 25 to 35 minutes. You might have to take them out every five minutes and stir up the mix to prevent burning.

The goal is to create an even golden brown or have them reach that lightly toasted color. Once you have got that, remove them from the oven.

Allow to cool and break them up and store in an airtight container.

Ketogenic Breakfast Burrito

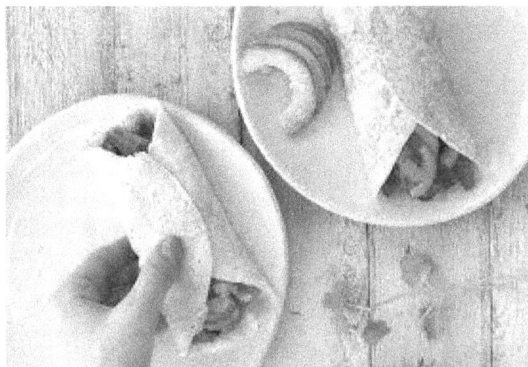

Total time: 20 minutes

Ingredients :

1 tbsp butter

2 eggs medium

2 tbsp full fat cream

choice of herbs or spices

salt and pepper to taste

Directions:

Grab a bowl and whisk the eggs and cream together. Add your choice of herbs and spices, depending on personal preferences.

Melt the butter in a frying pan using low to medium heat.

Pour the egg mixture into the pan.

Cook and swirl to create a thin layer of egg burrito.

Gently lift the egg burrito from the frying pan. Put the fillings you want inside and roll it up. Enjoy!

Baked lamb ribs macadamia with tomato salsa

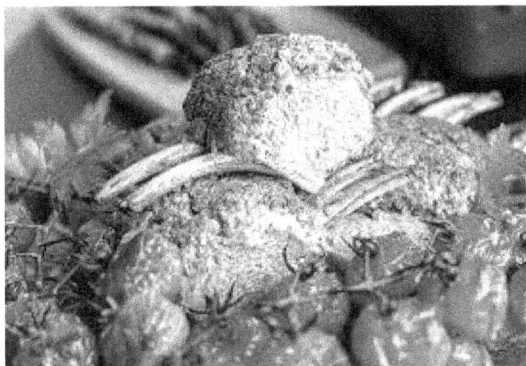

Total time: 45 minutes

Ingredients :

½ pound of fresh lamb ribs

½ cup of cherry tomatoes

½ teaspoon pepper

½ cup of macadamia

½ tablespoon of macadamia oil

¼ cup fresh parsley

1 teaspoon of balsamic vinegar

1 teaspoon of minced garlic

2 tablespoons of extra virgin olive oil

Directions

Cut up the lamb ribs into stripes or pieces

Preheat your oven to 204°C. Ensure that your baking tray is lined with aluminum foil.

Place the macadamia, garlic, parsley, pepper, and olive oil, in the food processor. Blend till the mixture is smooth and lump free.

Rub your processed mixture all over your cut lamb pieces. Ensure that it is coated well enough.

Arrange your strips nicely in the baking tray and bake for 20-25 minutes.

While the lamb bakes, cut the cherry in pieces. You can cut each into four then place them in an aluminum cup.

Pour macadamia oil on the tomatoes. Use spoon to mix the oil and tomatoes without squishing it. The aim is to get the oil all over it.

Take out your lamp and place on a plate.

Place your tomatoes in the oven for 4-5 minutes.

Take out the tomatoes and pour sparse amounts of balsamic vinegar and stir.

Pour the tomatoes on the lamb and serve warm.

Grilled Garlic Butter Shrimp

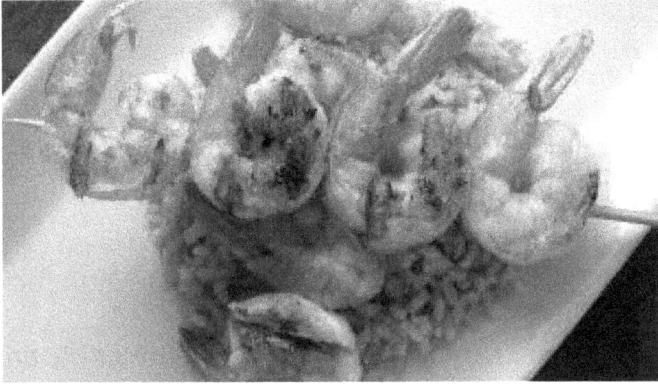

Total time: 35 minutes

Ingredients :

1 pound of large shrimps

1¼ tablespoon of minced garlic

1 teaspoon minced parsley, minced

½ cup of butter

Salt and pepper

Bamboo skewers

Directions

Defreeze, peel, and devein the shrimp. Be careful not to take off the tails.

Preheat the grill to medium heat. This should be around 360°F

Melt your butter.

Mix the melted butter with garlic. Add salt and pepper to your taste.

Put your bamboo skewers through the shrimp

Once grill is heated, place the shrimp on it and start cooking. Turn the shrimp over after 2 minutes.

Spread your garlic and butter mixture on the side facing you.

After two minutes, turn it over and spread the garlic and butter mix on the other side

After you have flipped the shrimp, baste the side facing up with the garlic butter sauce.

Ensure both sides are evenly cooked.

Remove the shrimp and serve

Tomato Chili Chicken Tender with Fresh Basils

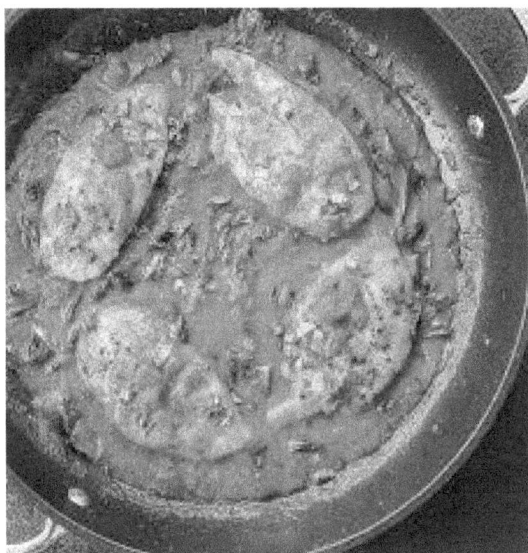

Total time: 50 minutes

Ingredients :

2 pounds of boneless chicken thighs

4 tablespoons extra virgin olive oil

3 lemon grasses

3 tablespoons red chili flakes

2½ tablespoons minced garlic

2 cups water

¼ cup sliced red tomatoes

½ cup fresh basils

Salt and pepper

Directions

Defreeze your chicken

Cut the chicken into small to medium pieces

Place the pieces in a skillet

Add some minced garlic and lemon grass

Add some salt and pepper to taste

Pour water over the chicken

Boil the chicken till the water totally/almost totally evaporates

Take out the chicken and set it aside

Heat a saucepan and pour olive oil in

Place the chicken and let it cook till it is brown

Place your tomatoes, basils, and chili flakes

Serve warm

Pork crack slaw

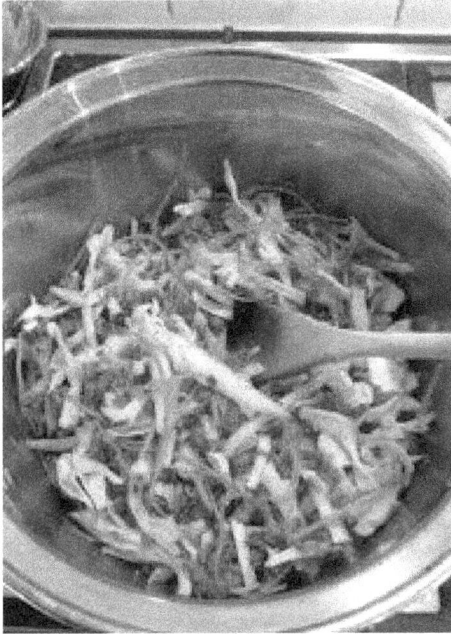

Total time: 30 minutes

Ingredients :

1 pound of ground pork sausage

1 teaspoon of mixed garlic

1 Bags of ready-mix dry coleslaw

1 teaspoon of sesame oil

2 tablespoons of rice vinegar

¼ of a red onion

¼ tablespoons of ground ginger

Salt and pepper to taste

Directions

Place the sausage in a bowl and heat till brown and ready, place in chopped red onions while you heat

When the sausage is ready, pour in the rice vinegar, sesame oil, minced garlic, coleslaw kits and salt and pepper to taste.

Stir on fore for five to seven minutes to enable everything cook

Pour in the soy sauce and cover the pot.

Let the contents steam for 5 to ten minutes

While it steams, dice half or a green onion and slice the other half to serve

Take it out and serve warm

Ketogenic lasagna

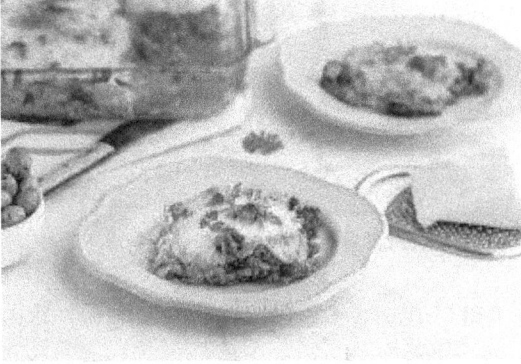

Total time: 30 minutes

Ingredients :

16 ounces of ricotta

8 ounces block cream cheese

4 cups of shredded mozzarella

4 minced cloves of garlic

3 large eggs

2 cups of freshly grated Parmesan cheese

1 tablespoon of extra virgin olive oil

1 ½ tablespoons of tomato paste

1 ½ ground beef

¾ cups of marinara

½ white or yellow onion

1 tablespoon of dried oregano

Cooking spray, butter, or oil

Pinch crushed red pepper flakes

Chopped parsley

Black pepper

Kosher salt

Directions

Preheat the oven to about 350° F

Lay a cooing parchment or foil on a large baking sheet and grease with cooking oil, or butter.

In another bowl, put in 2 ½ cups of mozzarella, 8 ounces of cheese, and 1 cup of parmesan cheese. Put in all the eggs and mix very well. Add salt and pepper to taste.

Pour on the baking sheet and spread it out

Bake for 15-20 minutes till its golden

Heat some oil in large skillet

Place chopped onion and fry it until it is soft

Add the garlic after and cook for a few more minutes

Poor in tomato paste

Heat the mixture until it is hot enough

Add salt and pepper to taste

Pour in ground beef

Cook the mixture until the meat loses its pink color

Add marinara

Put in red pepper flakes.

Cut noodles in 6 pieces.

Pour in a small amount of the sauce into a baking pan.

Then, put 2 noodles at the base. Divide the ricotta into 3. Spread one part of the ricotta over the broken noodles. Spread another part on the remaining meat and sauce which is on the top. Pour in a last part with the parmesan cheese. Make similar layers and pour cheese at the very top.

Place the mix in the oven until the cheese melts and the sauce heats

Sprinkle parsley and cheese if you wish

Easy meal prep chicken soup

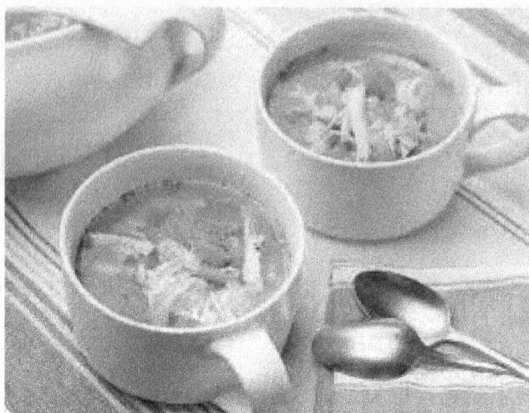

Total time: 45 minutes

Ingredients :

15 chicken breast tenderloins

2 tablespoons garlic powder

1 cup of chopped carrots

1 cup of chopped celery

1 tablespoon butter

Salt

Black pepper

Directions

Unfreeze chicken breast tenderloins

Place in put with 1 ½ cups of water.

Put it a teaspoon of salt

Put in ½ teaspoon of black pepper

94

Put in 1 tablespoon of garlic

Let the chicken boil for 20-25 minutes till soft and almost ready

Put in chopped carrots and chopped celery

Put in another tablespoon of garlic

Put in butter and cover for 5 to 10 minutes

You can freeze till needed and simply reheat when you need it.

Ketogenic burger

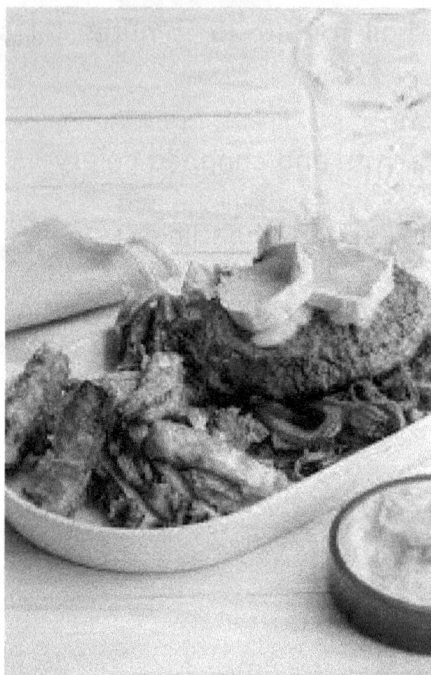

Total time: 50 minutes

Ingredients :

4 pounds of ground hamburger meat

8 tablespoons of half melted butter

5 cloves of garlic, minced

4 tablespoons Worcestershire sauce

1 teaspoon of ground black pepper

1 tablespoon of salt

Directions

Put in the meat, sauce, pepper, and garlic. Put in salt to taste.

Mix the ingredients very well with a big spoon.

Pour out the mixture on a clean board and mold into discs. Use that shape to form the mixture into patties

Put a tablespoon of butter in the center of each patty

Mold the butter into each patty

Place on a grill. Cook each side for around seven minutes

You can try cooking these burgers in foil to prevent it from catching fire due to the increased fat levels

Calamari mayo with cauliflower broccoli salad

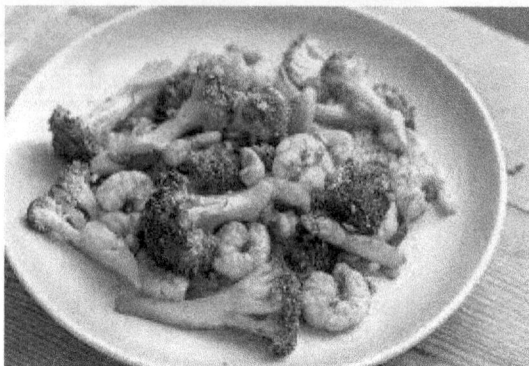

Total time: 35 minutes

Ingredients :

1 ½ pounds of fresh squids

1 ½ tablespoons of lemon juice

2 eggs

2 cups of almond flour

2 cups of broccoli florets

2 cups of cauliflower florets

1 cup of extra virgin olive oil

1 diced onion

½ cup diced cheddar cheese

½ cup of mayonnaise

½ teaspoon of pepper

½ cup of sour cream

Directions

Steam cauliflower and broccoli until they are soft and tender

Place them in bowl for later use

Remove squid ink

Crack eggs

Add salt and pepper to eggs for taste

Cut the squid into rings

Put the squid in the egg mix

Pour in almond flour

Rub in the flour into the squid and egg mix

Heat a pan and pour in oil

Fry the squid in oil until it is golden brown

Take out the squid from the oil and set it aside

In a separate bowl, put in mayonnaise, lemon juice, and sour cream

Mix well

To serve, place the fried squid on a plate with the steam broccoli and cauliflower florets then drip the mayonnaise, lemon juice, and sour cream on it

Sprinkle dry cheddar cheese

Ketogenic strawberry rice

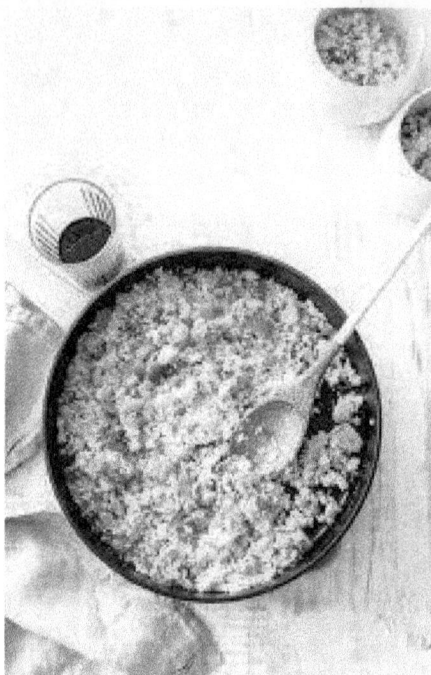

Total time: 40 minutes

Ingredients :

3 cups of sliced strawberries

Cinnamon

2 cups of cooked rice

2 tablespoons of grass-fed butter

2 cup full-fat organic coconut milk

1 tablespoon of pure vanilla extract

½ cup birch xylitol

Himalayan pink salt

¼ teaspoon ground

Directions

Put your 2 ½ cups of sliced strawberries, cinnamon, cooked rice, grass-fed butter, full-fat organic coconut milk, pure vanilla extract, birch xylitol, and a pinch of salt in a saucepan

Cook for 2-30 minutes while stirring till it becomes creamy

Cut up the remaining strawberries

Place the cut-up berries on the rice mixture and serve warm

Ketogenic white rice

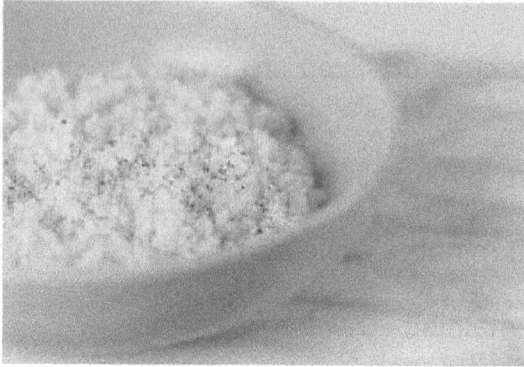

Total time: 65 minutes

Ingredients :

1 cup of rice

1 cup of diced tomatoes

1 ¼ cups of diced peppers

Extra virgin olive oil ½ cup

½ cup of boiled ground beef

1/8 cup of diced green onions

1/8 cup of sliced spring onions

Salt

Adobo seasoning

Directions

Put 3-4 cups of water in a large saucepan and bring to boil

Put in your rice when it starts to boil and put in a tablespoon of salt

After 16-20 minutes, the rice should be ready. If you are not quite sure, you can fish it for a grain or three to taste

There should still be lots of water in the pot and so, you should strain it out. Straining the water drains out some of the starch which means you reduce the carbs. You can use a strainer with tiny holes.

Place your strained rice in a pot and cover.

Preheat your saucepan

Pour in your extra virgin oil and let it heat very slightly

Pour in your diced green onions. Fry for 15 seconds. While frying, stir it so it does not burn

Put in your spring onions and fry for another 15 seconds. Remember to stir.

Put in your pepper and stir for half a minute

Put in your tomatoes and stir.

Stir together for 5-7 minutes

Put in your boiled ground beef

Put in a teaspoon of salt

Put in a teaspoon of Adobo seasoning

Stir together for 5-8 minutes

Place your boiled rice in a serving dish.

Spread your sauce over the rice.

Enjoy hot or warm

Steamed veggies and prawn with coconut milk

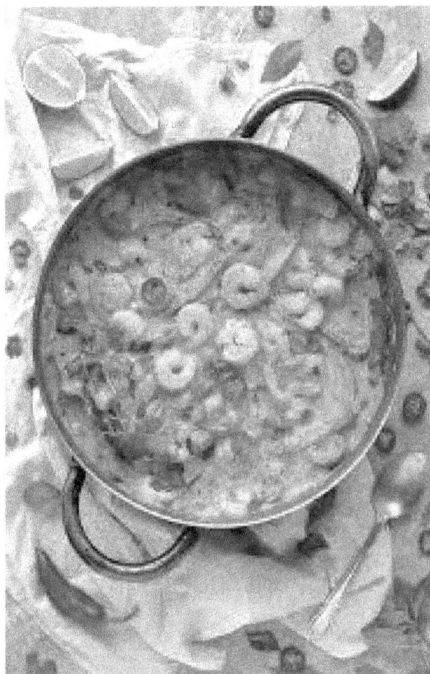

Total time: 45 minutes

Ingredients :

1 pound of fresh shrimps

4 tablespoons of extra virgin olive oil

1 egg

1/8 cup of coconut milk

½ cup almond flour

¼ cup water

1/8 of cup grated cheddar cheese

1/8 cup of diced carrot

1/8 of cup diced onion

1/8 of cup chopped leek

Directions

Peel prawns, remove heads and set aside

Crack a mix an egg in a bowl

Mix water and almond flour with water

Pour in half of the egg

Mix with a spoon

Use the mixture to make omelets

Take your peeled prawns and put them in a food processor

Process till smooth

Preheat a skillet

Pour in 1 ½ spoons of the olive oil

Put in onion and sauté. Stir fry till it is golden brown

Add the leak and carrot and stir for ten seconds

Pour in coconut milk

Stir till the milk disappears

Put the cooked veggies, prawns, and remaining half egg into the bowl

Mix well

Put an omelet on a plate and put a tablespoon of the prawn mix

Fold the omelet like an envelope

Repeat with the rest of the omelets

Preheat a saucepan and then pour the remaining olive oil into it.

When the oil is a bit hot, put the prawn envelopes in the saucepan

Cook for 2 minutes on each side till golden brown

Serve warm

Mediterranean pork chops

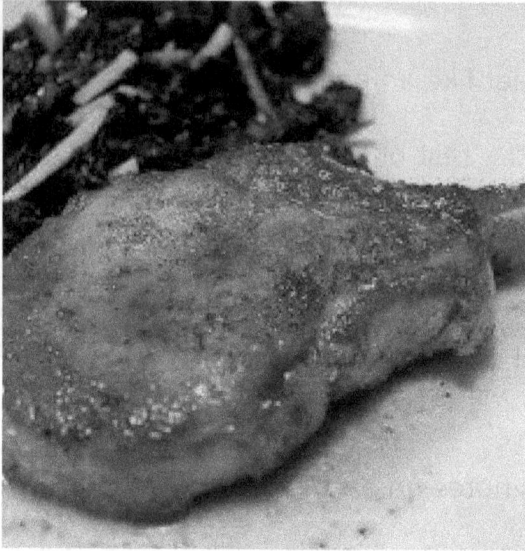

Total time: 45 minutes

Ingredients :

8 boneless pork loin chops

1 teaspoon of black pepper

1 teaspoon of kosher salt

7 minced garlic cloves

2 tablespoons of chopped and fresh rosemary

Directions

Mix garlic and rosemary in a bowl

Place pork chops in a bowl. Sprinkle pepper and salt

Rub in the salt and pepper

Rub in garlic and rosemary

Place pork chops in roasting pan at 425 degrees F. Do this for ten minutes

Reduce the temperature of the oven to 350 F degrees and continue roasting for about 20-25 minutes

Serve warm